TRAUMA I

MW00935283

The Revolutionary Step-By-Step Program
for Eliminating Effects of Childhood Abuse,
Trauma, Emotional Pain and Crippling Inner Stress, to
Living in Joy without Drugs or Therapy

ANNE MARGOLIS
CNM, LM, MSN, BSN, RNC

DEDICATION

This book is dedicated to those who are done suffering and are ready to heal and create a life they love. It is dedicated to those who want to live fully and vibrantly.

It is dedicated to those who want to take themselves and others higher, no matter what it takes, despite the occasional setbacks, who are willing to play full out, and plow forward despite the fears.

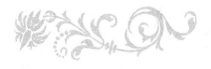

ACKNOWLEDGEMENTS

I want to thank my dear beloved friend and colleague Dr. Barbara Gordon Cohen for being with me through it all, always inspiring me to heal, laugh, play, travel and do retreats together. She taught me the meaning of true friendship and sisterhood, staying with me through the night of my worst darkness.

I want to thank my husband Jay, for really being there with me always, like a solid mountainous rock in every storm, and every sunshine, devoted, giving, loving and adoring, supporting me when others doubted, believing in me, proud of me — who I became given what I had been through.

I want to thank my children, such dear beautiful souls, for everything they do and who they are, and for being my most profound gurus.

I am humbly grateful to God for my gifts and my blessings, and also for all the challenges and hardships I endured, as they made me who I am today.

I want to thank Lucy Hamel — who midwifed me through my first rebirthing breathwork session that began the journey of saving my life. I will always remember her wise soul, her kind heart, her provocative transformative activities she led in our personal and group workshop sessions, her playfulness, and her friendship. I thank Patsy Brennan, who guided many of my breathwork sessions with devotion and heart, and saw me in my divine magnificence and strength, beyond my self limiting thoughts and beliefs that simply were not at all true. We became such friends — talking and laughing for hours —- beyond the breath. She inspired me to write this book to inspire others.

I am eternally grateful for my teachers and founders of Clarity Breathwork — Ashanna Solaris and Dana Dharma Devi Delong — living goddesses. Words cannot express my gratitude for all they have done for me and the other souls so blessed to have been touched by them. They are truly healing the world and are a huge source of powerful light — with a rippling effect beyond what any of us could fathom.

I am so thankful to have had the opportunity to take and assist at their incredible workshops, and have had many private sessions with them both. When I find gold I must share it and keep connected to it. They are pure gold. I tell everyone about them and their work — I want to shout out from the rooftops so all those who need it access the healing that is their birthright, which is why I do what I do and am writing this book.

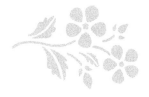

They guided me to release billions of tons of trapped trauma energy in my body never to return, and reset my suffering nervous system. I am still amazed by the miracles I experienced. I got myself back — the playful powerful ball of joy and love that I am. I found a global community of like minded sisters and brothers for which have created and hold safe loving space. This healing was so palpable people notice and my relationships and just about every aspect of my life improved immensely. I was so blown away by my recovery I had to become a practitioner and help others find this relief, deep healing, clarity, forgiveness, and return to themselves and their joy.

I know my healing comes from the profound power of the Breathwork, but it was so much more. It was facilitated by their beautiful music and meditations like no other, by the community dancing, the group interactions and activities they lead us through, by the sensitive, loving, compassionate and open environment they create, their sincere passion for this work, their authenticity.

And it was not just me. I was amazed by the healing I witnessed and similar feelings expressed by the other participants in every group I was blessed to be a part of.

I will forever sing their praises.

Lastly, I must thank Regena Thomashauer, Mama Gena and her School of Womanly Arts, for her brilliance, her boldness, her outrageousness and her courage, for believing in me, pushing my edges way passed my comfort zone, for empowering me to own my divine feminine gifts and my voice, for helping me to return to myself and my rapturous sensual joy, love, laughter, fun and play - so key to healing and living fully, for giving me space to be myself, shine, lead and inspire others, and dance like no one is watching — for pure joy and celebration, and for moving my emotions, all of which I have come to embrace. Her teachings have transformed my life and my relationships and my work. I bring them everywhere. I want to thank dear souls and total inspirations Lauren Abrami, and Bernadette Pleasant, as well as the rest of the entire devoted staff, the sisterhood they all create, and for the opportunity to be on Team Pleasure, giving back as a volunteer. They all helped me to recover my life, live fully and vibrantly. I am eternally grateful for that and so much more.

Each and everyone of you, and the HUGE healing I experienced, are in my gratitude practice every day, and it brings me to tears thinking about it and how I got myself and my life back beyond my wildest dreams, from the pits of hopeless agony.

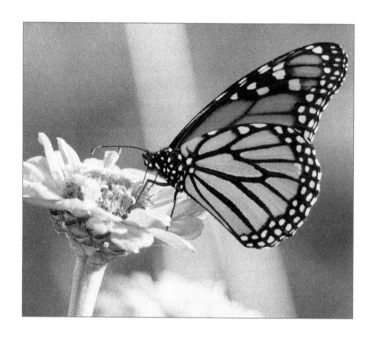

"*I want to thank my children, such dear beautiful souls, for everything they do and who they are, and for being my most profound gurus.*"

FOREWORD

Anne Margolis has been a dear colleague, close friend of mine, and more like a soulmate since we met more than 25 years ago. We were neighbors and clicked right away, having similar backgrounds and interests. We were busy living our lives unconsciously going through our routines of working, having children and raising a family. We are both in healing professions — Anne as a Holistic Midwife/OB/GYN Nurse Practitioner, Yoga Teacher and Certified Clarity Breathwork Practitioner and myself as an Integrative Osteopath Physician — and were were taking care of everyone else, but ourselves. We awoke gradually, and began to journey together into consciousness by traveling to Costa Rica, the Caribbean and Kripalu Center in Massachusetts, for rest and relaxation, yoga, massage, and rebirthing breathwork retreats and workshops both in search of becoming more peaceful within to face some of the greatest life challenges to help ourselves, families and patients. We needed to take breaks from the intensity of our lives, exploring, living fully, laughing, being ourselves, and healing. Our vacations together became necessities. We took off from our hectic work schedules, as we planned, coveted and guarded them with care.

Ahhhh....the taste of freedom, joy, fun and play; recharging and restoring, the warm sun and beauty of the tropical Caribbean. We fell apart together and literally helped each other through our processes. We have been there for each other in tough times and great times and our healing continues together no matter where we are. We have been through a lot together navigating our way as holistic health care professionals and mothers.

Anne worked as part of my staff in my Integrative medical practice , as a nurse practitioner and midwife for many years. We shared a common interest in nutrition, acupuncture, homeopathy, yoga, breath work, massage, meditation, and osteopathy. We both drew on a variety of alternative modalities to help ourselves and clients heal such as Dr. Sarno's method for healing pain, Imago therapy, biofeedback, and The Journey work. She advocated for a number of women sexually abused by a member of high clergy who sought her guidance — despite being threatened, she was instrumental in the pursuit of effective justice. I marvel as she helps thousands of women and their families around the world along their journeys to giving birth, teaching yoga for pregnancy and beyond, assisting in the natural process of pregnancy, birth and postpartum and guiding Clarity Breathwork sessions with her gentle hands, intuitive wisdom, and beautiful soul.

Anne has endured many of life's enormous challenges, including severe child abuse and abandonment, having a child with a life-threatening illness who survived a bone marrow transplant donated by another one of her children, pressures from practicing midwifery, living in a family and community that had very different cultural and religious lifestyles from her own and committed to keeping her family together, rooted and stable…to name just a few. She has become quite an empowered and inspiring woman who can now use her voice to create a beautiful life for herself and others. She has come into her authentic being and is doing what she really wants to do in life and living every moment with her love, passion, and light shining through. She has learned to navigate the difficulties in her life with positivity, gratitude, and joy.

Anne is involved every step of the way in assisting you to heal emotional wounds and allowing your vessel to be completely free of repressed inner childhood and adult pain as well guiding you in pregnancy, labor and postpartum. Her book is transformative and empowering. A must read!

~ *Dr. Barbara Gordon-Cohen, D.O., Integrative Medical Practitioner*
Author of Bridging the Gap to Oneness:
Dr. Barbara's Integrative Guide to Healing and Wholeness
www.DoctorBarbara.com

A MESSAGE FROM THE CO-CREATOR OF CLARITY BREATHWORK

In my 25-plus years as a healer and facilitator of others, I have found the most important key to healing is in the power of our very own Breath. Most of us don't breathe fully. We hold our breath and may have been holding it since the first breath, if the cord was cut too soon and we were held upside down and spanked. Welcome to the World!

Many of us experienced trauma at our births due to unconscious birthing practices. We were not able to bond fully with our mothers and experience true connection, which is our mammalian birthright. As a result, the vast majority of us experience some degree of loneliness, despair, longing for something we cannot name, a sense of disconnection and suffer from a wide range of depression and anxiety symptoms. Antidepressants and addictions are widespread as a way to escape this pain, and yet bring their own host of side effects and never seem to get at the root of the real issue and transform it.

There is another way!

I've been fortunate enough to lead thousands of people through the profound practice of Clarity Breathwork, which I pioneered and co-founded with Dana DeLong. Together, we have witnessed incredible miracles of healing, integration, completion of old wounds and supporting people to open to a greater sense of feeling connected to themselves, others, the World and the greater mysterious cosmos that we are a part of.

We are delighted that Anne Margolis — nurse, midwife — was able to use this work to transform years of abuse and challenges in her life. There is no one better suited than someone who has welcomed thousands of babies into the world and understands the intricacies of birth to help you re-birth yourself as life intended you to be: open, free and experiencing greater joy and ease in every area of your life. She is a wonderful example that healing is not only possible, it is inevitable when we find the right pathway to support ourselves.

Anne has supported our trainings in Costa Rica and Mt. Shasta and brings an incredible presence of unconditional love, compassion and expertise in the unraveling of trauma and opening to more joy!

Our amazing graduate and practitioner Anne Margolis, is sharing the Breath in New York and now globally! With her decades long background as a midwife, she is totally rockin' it with Clarity Breathwork, sending ripples of transformation and healing out far and wide.

Thank you, Anne!

~ *Ashanna Solaris, co-founder of Clarity Breathwork*
www.ashannasolaris.com
www.claritybreathwork.com

INTRODUCTION

Rebirthing yourself after trauma can mean total healing, when we learn to embrace the trauma as a transitional life lesson, rather than a life sentence, and when we learn the keys to healing and transforming our suffering. The idea for this book was birthed from my own trauma and my experiences with others who have endured pain and agony on their road to wellness. I am actually grateful for my own story of trauma and abuse as it made me who I am today. As a midwife, I help babies and their parents birth, and as a Certified Clarity Breathwork Practitioner. I help people rebirth themselves, heal their wounds and suffering, reclaim their inner peace and joy that is all of our birth right.

Thank you for reading this book, and please feel free to contact me to learn more about how you, too, can finally be 100 percent free from the imprints and impacts of trauma. I had a great childhood, a loving doting family and extended family, and was the only grandchild on both sides. I was a ball of energy, enthusiasm, joy, laughter, fun and play — and I lit up the room wherever I entered. My world was glorious. Then things changed. I will share a glimpse of a much larger story, so you can at least get a sense of what it was like to be me, why I am passionate about doing what I do, and see the healing possibilites for you as well.

~ *Anne Margolis*

ABOUT THE TRAUMA RELEASE FORMULA

If you've experienced intense stress, emotional pain or any type of trauma, this program is a must - it represents sincere hope that saved my life and the lives of countless others. Once you know the key that unlocks the emotional pain, suffering, your ongoing personal life, work and relationship issues, and chronic stress related physical symptoms and illness, and how to unlock it all, you experience such huge relief and a powerful healing. I would say just about everyone has baggage, past trauma of some sort, emotional pain and inner stress that is part of being human. Or it comes out as physical problems.

This book is designed to help you release trauma through dealing with each negative experience in a step-by-step process that allows the gentle tuning of your body, to the original state it was in before the trauma occurred. Stay strong as you work through the lessons in this book and know there is hope on the other side. Using breathwork, emotionally expressive dance, non-traditional methods of moving trauma and total self-acceptance — you will see healing, almost instantly.

"The wound is the place where the Light enters you." ∽ *Rumi*

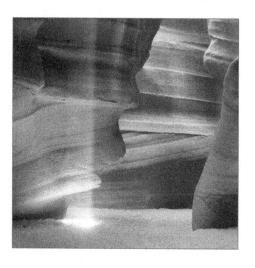

CONTENTS

CONTENTS

MY PERSONAL TRAUMA STORY

How I Healed My Life

For more than 22 years, I have worked as a holistic nurse midwife, and many years as a yoga teacher, advanced graduate and volunteer staff of Mama Gena's School of Womanly Arts, and a Certified Clarity Breathwork practitioner. I have shared the most intimate experiences with women and their families as they move from being teenagers through adulthood, parenting, and aging.

I have held space for the huge powerful transformation of birth — that involves challenging situations of extreme intensity, vulnerability, pain of all degrees, facing enormous fears head on, surrendering to a process far greater than all of us that helps create enormous joy, love, and miracles.

Over many years, the women in my practice, their partners, extended families and friends have shared with me and sought my guidance for their deepest darkest sufferings. I would say just about everyone has baggage, past trauma of some sort, emotional pain, and inner stress that is part of being human. It comes out as emotional pain, or it comes out as physical problems.

There is no pain — physical or emotional — that scares me — I am comfortable with it all; I have either felt it myself, witnessed it, and helped others move through and heal from it.

I know that we as divine human beings can get through just about anything. You are incredibly resilient — no matter how extreme a trauma you endured. Your are bigger than any fear, resistance, or memory, you are bigger than any pain. You can absolutely normalize and reset entrenched dysfunctional response patterns, no matter how severe the trauma.

Everything Changed

I had a great childhood, loving family and extended family. My world was glorious. I was an enthusiastic ball of light, joy, play, laughter....then everything changed. I was 9, when my mom lost her mom (my nana) at a young age, quickly, aggressively and painfully to cancer. My mom became very dark, angry and scary, and snapped into what I now know to be a serious mental illness called BPD (borderline personality disorder). I never imagined such crippling hopeless despair of a helpless victim I needed to rescue, alternating with the conniving terrifying rage of a witch from whom I had to escape. And, then sometimes I got a glimpse of my loving mother. I walked on eggshells as I never knew who she would be or what she would do.

Around this time, the screaming started, at me and my Dad, and then the abuse. Terrible abuse. My dad and extended family were my haven. But little by little, they moved far away. They had no tools to deal with the horror but to deny, neglect, escape and abandon. My dad was a busy doctor, but when he could, he would take me on day trips and weekend getaways. He played all sorts of games with me. I loved and felt so comforted by my dad, and I cherished those special times we had together. When he wasn't home, it could be pure terror.

I don't have much memory of my adolescence and teen-aged years, but there is one key episode that is vivid in my mind.

One day, my dad took me in his arms and said he loved me very much, but was so sorry — he could not live in the house with my mom anymore, and had to leave. He planned to live with a new lady he now loved. He was leaving me to go live with her and her three children, four hours away.

"You can always come visit," he said. My world tumbled down around me. I clinged to his ankles, sobbing, begging and pleading for him not to leave. He picked up his suitcases, and walked out of the front door. He was gone: Forever.

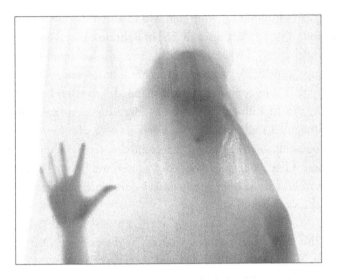

Mom said she loved me. Dad said he loved me. They all said they loved me — but that "love" came with the severe pain of abuse, abandonment, neglect, the huge loss of my roots, sense of safety, and trust. All of my core needs as a child were blown up and destroyed leaving me with no solid foundation. At the time, my baby sister was only 8 months old, and I knew I had to protect her, too. I had to grow up fast.

My mother committed much of her life to revenge and to ruining my dad. I was not allowed to see him or his family, or even some members of my mother's family that she felt hurt by, as she said they were plotting evil against us and seeing them would betray her. Of course, I had to see them, so I had to sneak out and lie, all while my insides were on fire. Against my will, I also had to do and say things for my mom for the court case, or face her terrifying wrath.

I disassociated, buried, repressed and escaped from it all — what most young teens do — and delved into school work, after-school jobs, team sports, dance, guitar, my friends, and as I got older my steady boyfriend. I prayed to God, (I did not know was there) to rescue me.

It was no surprise, I was a young bride. Just out of college, I married a kind, trustworthy, stable, principled man who adored me and had a loving family.

As an adult, I did not remember feeling good, or at ease, and I continued to bury myself in busyness to not feel the discomfort and pain inside. I had one huge stress event or trauma after another.

My own "birth trauma story" stands out to me.

My Birth Trauma Story

I was 24 and an OB Nurse working in a typical community hospital when I first became pregnant. It was not expected or planned, I was in no way ready to be a mother, but I loved this baby growing in me with all my heart and soul, and I made an unspoken vow from the depths of my being, which was that I would never ever do to her or any of my future children what my parents had done to me. I never broke my vow.

You'd think I'd have been prepared for labor and delivery, but working in the hospital is where I developed my strong fear of birth in the first place!

My family and friends didn't live near me. I didn't know people in my neighborhood where we lived for my husband's work; and I didn't know about doulas or midwives. I felt so alone. I had a lot of fear of birth; and I was really afraid of all the things I witnessed in the hospital as an obstetric (OB) nurse – especially of having major abdominal surgery and that something would go really wrong. I didn't trust birth, the professionals, or myself.

I had no sense that pregnancy and birth were normal and beautiful. As a nurse on the unit, I was given the royal treatment. But it did not feel that way in my body.

I wish I could say that my own birth trauma story is an exception, but unfortunately, it's a common experience still today. I hear it from thousands of women. In most hospitals in the United States, labor is looked at as a catastrophe or disaster waiting to happen, resulting in a potential lawsuit. Childbirth, in the hospital where I worked, felt like an emergency or intensive care situation the majority of the time. It was also like I was working in a factory: get em in, get em out and I saw a lot of crises. There was no calm, no beauty, no joy, no humanity, no concern for individuals, or their feelings. It was about expecting the worst and maintaining protection from litigation. That was my experience.

I was actually in more operating rooms than delivery rooms, and I was assisting more cesarean births than I ever thought I would. I was having to rescue women and babies from complications caused by routine medical interventions. It scared me not just as a pregnant mother, but even more as a nurse. And, this is where birth trauma begins: chronic fear and inner stress are the enemies of childbirth. If a birthing mother is feeling stressed and afraid, she will not labor well, especially if her feelings go unheard and are disregarded. She will need interventions that lead to more problems and a cascade of more interventions.

At the time, I thought this was standard operating procedure. I didn't know what was missing. I just knew it was scary. My hands were tied as a nurse. I didn't trust birth or myself, and because of what I saw as a nurse, I did not trust the doctor or hospital either. My obstetrician was a nice man, my colleague, but the vibes during the short office visits with him were cold, impersonal, and alarming. Even though I often told my doctor that I felt worried and scared, my feelings were dismissed, as though they were unimportant and irrelevant. I started to think something was wrong with me.

> *"There was no calm, no beauty,*
> *no joy, no humanity."*

My stress only increased from there. When I went into labor, one of the first things I had to do when I got to the hospital was take off my own clothes, and put on a hospital gown. It seemed innocuous then – what we all did. I look back on that now and see the disempowerment and depersonalization. A hospital gown creates a sense of vulnerability, a feeling of being sick, dependent, and becoming an assembly line patient. It just felt wrong: I wasn't a patient, I wasn't sick — I was a birthing mother in labor; I did not know there were options.

I had to lie down in bed, even though I wanted to stand; my body needed to do move around, but I had to stay still, so the nurse and doctor could read the monitors placed on me. When a mom is in labor, her body assumes a natural upright mobile position. It only makes sense — to get your baby to come down and out through your pelvis and vaginal canal, gravity is your friend! The pelvis is three bones connected by ligaments. The pelvic diameter is smaller when lying flat on your back, but can stretch and move to accommodate baby when it is in other more upright and asymmetrical positions.

I was attached to an IV and told not to eat food or drink. I know now, like any athlete — if you were about do any long and hard physical activity, like running the 26-mile marathon, it's never recommended to go without oral fuel and hydration.

My doctor didn't talk to me much or explain things. He just kept giving me frequent internal exams without even asking, then telling the results to the nurse outside my room. "She's still 4," he kept saying. Finally, I heard, "Hang Pit." As a nurse — I know what that was. I was familiar with the procedures, I knew they were going to give me the medication Pitocin and that it would cause my contractions to come more frequently, and to become much longer and harder than they naturally would.

When I said, "No, I did not want Pit." I remember my nurse's well-meaning response as she was putting the medicine in my IV. She said, "Honey, you don't want a cesarean to do you?"

"I was so young and afraid, and I did not feel safe or secure."

It was either take the medication, or be faced with the possibility of a C-section. (I did not know what I know now, that these weren't my only two options and that my body was capable.) Of course, I did not want a cesarean, major abdominal surgery, so I agreed.

I felt feared into it. At that point, my Lamaze training went out the window. I was in unnecessary highly intense pain, and I couldn't handle the agony brought on by the medication. The doctor came in and walked out again. He said, "She's still at a 4. Give her an epidural."

It seemed like forever, and then they were giving me an epidural anesthetic via a big needle into my back, the area around my spinal cord.

I was so young and afraid, and I did not feel safe or secure. My feelings were totally overlooked, no one seemed to hear what I wanted and needed, and all of the things that came naturally were discouraged. I had no sense of control over my own body or birth. And, then I went numb from the waist down.

My Worst Fear Happened

Suddenly, my worst fear happened. There was a serious and prolonged drop in my baby's heart rate from the medication. There was a panic in the room. The doctor told the alarmed staff to prepare for an emergency/stat cesarean. They had minutes to get my baby out. I had seen so many bad things happen to women and babies in this process. I was rolled away on a stretcher in a frenzy, and then was left alone in the operating room on the operating table, after they scrubbed me down, waiting for the assistant surgeon who never came.

I was watching the clock. Ten, 20 , 30, 45, 60 minutes passed.

No one was monitoring me or my baby. For an hour, I was completely alone, even my husband was not allowed in the room. At first, I was convinced my baby was severely damaged from lack of oxygen, but then dead by now. At some point the meds took over my body, I started pushing. I called for help. The doctor ran in yelling, "Get me a vacuum." He cut a big episiotomy and put strong suction on her head and vacuumed my daughter out vaginally.

I didn't want to see her because I believed that by now I would be looking at her dead body. They reassured me that she was just fine and told me to look. She was pink, breathing, healthy, and appreared vigorous. I was still too afraid to look at her. They said again, she was fine. She was beautiful.

But, I was not fine. I was traumatized.

I had what I now know to be birth trauma. PTSD (posttraumatic stress disorder) is a normal response to such an intense horrific situation. I had the symptoms, I just did not know what was wrong at the time. I was getting frequent flashbacks of the experience, anything that reminded me of the birth triggered horrible symptoms in my body; I had a fight or flight response whenever I saw a pregnant woman or new baby, or whenever anyone would ask me about my birth or talk about their birth – I could not discuss any of it without feeling awful inside. I was wound up tight like a spring, hyper-alert, overprotective, and worried something terrible would happen to her. I was getting panic attacks, and I couldn't sleep.

Even though I loved her completely and whole heartedly, she was so beautiful and innocent, it was hard to look at her and not be reminded of the birth experience, and to feel triggered into a panic. I could not even imagine going back to work and facing the scene. I began having nightmares. My adrenaline would pump up, and I would feel sick. I'd was on-guard all of the time, because I was also afraid of the intolerable sensations in my body.

> *"We live in a society that tends to repress feelings, and that's what I did."*

"You'll get over it," well-meaning people would say; or they would ask me, "What is the big deal? You have a healthy baby." That made me feel worse, like something was really wrong with me, so I felt more ashamed, alone, and isolated. I stopped telling anyone what I was feeling.

As a new mom experiencing birth trauma that I did not know I had, I sucked it up. We live in a society that tends to repress feelings, and that's what I did. People and medical professionals did not and often still do not take seriously the huge impact of birth on the psychology of women. I repressed and suppressed and tried my best to move on. I am amazed I was able to go back to work, but it was not easy.

I told my husband that I never wanted to have another baby.

It was no surprise, I became pregnant again two years later, and started having panic attacks. Also, I ended up having a very similar experience to my first birth, this time with a different doctor in the hospital.

I was telling a friend about my frustrations with the system and she told me I should become a midwife. I literally asked her, "What's a midwife?"

There was no internet or world wide web at that time. I went to the library to research it, and applied soon after. I was accepted to the oldest nurse-midwifery school in the country.

Midwifery started the journey of healing and coming home to myself.

I was in midwifery school during my third pregnancy. I was still traumatized from my two previous births, but I now knew what was possible. I hired an excellent midwife and looked forward to a much better experience the third-time around.

I prepared in a whole different way and I had a completely transformed mindset. My birth team, setting, preparation and mindset shift were keys to my success.

I told my midwife that for me to authentically practice midwifery, it had to work for me. Honestly, I really did not think I could actually do it. She reassured me I could, and that it would prove to be healing and empowering.

The experience was as different as night from day in comparison to my previous pregnancies and births.

In labor and birth, I wasn't tied down to the bed. It was a relaxed environment. I would labor in the tub, and in the shower. We played music and I would dance. She would periodically check my baby's heart rate. The birthing process was beautiful and was treated as something normal rather than a crisis. I wasn't left alone by my midwife. She helped me with her words and her heart, allowing my body to do what it was designed to do. She gave me the trust that my body could do it. I wasn't afraid. I felt very supported.

I wasn't an emergency room patient; I was a strong woman having a baby. It was challenging but so doable, I was encouraged to find my own strength and I did it! I was so proud of myself. It not only helped to begin to heal my birth trauma, it restored my confidence; it also convinced me that midwifery care works, and that I could now truly help women as a midwife. My fourth birth had all these same components and reinforced my awakening, my healing, and passion to help others have these kinds of experiences.

I was so relieved after my own last two births in this way, I was filled with elation beyond words. I experienced delicious, wonderful transformation and miracles. Every day and every moment I think about it, I am brought to tears of gratitude for this work, for all the living angels who guided me to this place.

As I got older and faced a lot of big stresses, and real traumas one after another, I just kept repressing and suppressing — it was subconscious — I mastered it as a kid. Over and over I got knocked down, but then I got up. I kept it all together.

I had by now a very busy midwifery practice and was raising four kids, but I was not feeling well inside. I was midwifing everyone, but myself.

The Wakeup Call

The main wake-up call was when my young teen-aged daughter was diagnosed with a serious life-threatening illness around the same time her best friend died from something similar.

We tried everything alternative and then conventional treatment modalities. The only treatment to save her life was a bone marrow transplant after high dose chemotherapy. One of my young children was the perfect match donor. My daughter miraculously recovered after eight years of hell. And her doctor, chief of Bone Marrow Transplant (BMT) at the hospital, came to her wedding.

But in the midst of it, everything just became too much. I had had enough. The mountain was too big. I had nothing left to fight it.

At one point, I fell to the floor writhing in deep emotional pain that just seemed to take over. I wept, and I prayed. I felt no one heard or answered. It was absolute torture to be in my body. I was finally ready to give into it. BUT — I knew I did not want to stay curled up into a fetal position. I did not want to be like my poor mother, who has lived her life as a powerless victim, lamenting over all the terrible things that happened to her.

You don't know how strong you are until you have to be that strong. I made a choice to do whatever it took to get myself well, to take myself higher to be there for myself, my family, my friends and the families in my practice. There was no other way. I upped my selfcare, improved my already healthy diet, took more dance classes, and tried just about everything — acupuncture, Journey work, hypnotherapy, massage, biofeedback, supplements, herbs, homeopathy, chiropractic and osteopathic care, and Reiki. I read piles of self-help books, went to numerous healing workshops and retreats. Nothing touched it — not even my more regular and deeper yoga and meditation practice.

I did all sorts of therapy with a variety of therapists — but talking about it and wallowing in the pain just made it worse.

I eventually went to doctors and psychiatrists who just wanted to drug me. I knew that was not the cure, but I was so desperate I tried a few. The side effects were even more intolerable, and no medication actually helped. Nothing worked. I was not far from giving up, but I couldn't give up. It is not my personality to give up.

Healing Begins

I searched for and found a holistic integrative psychiatrist who had a wonderful reputation and came highly recommended. I told her I was going crazy and something was terribly wrong. She spent more than 1 1/2 hours with me, and focused a lot on my childhood, about which I did not have much memory. She said I am not crazy. She nailed it. She said I had chronic PTSD (posttraumatic stress disorder), from adult traumas, but more significantly from the years of severe abuse I had experienced as a child through teen years during my most crucial formative development.

I had never used those words before to describe my past, but it made so much sense. She said all the remedies and treatments I had tried did not work because cutting edge trauma research indicates ***unprocessed trauma is stored as trapped energy in the body***, and it needs to be released from the body with somatic types of therapies — not even by talking about it or medication. My central nervous system needed to be reset, as it was in a perpetual state of self-preservation fight or flight, which causes dis-ease and many of the physical and mental health problems of modern living.

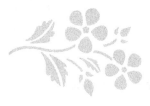

Trauma Release

Other medical professionals said I was so damaged, I would never heal. She said it was serious, but I absolutely could heal. I was thrilled to get a diagnosis and hope for a cure, and to hear I was not going nuts (even though it felt like it!). She mentioned trauma therapies like Somatic Experience (SE) and Organic Intelligence (OI), but first and foremost, I must follow a trauma release and nervous system reset regimen.

Then I needed empowerment, to get back my joy and play and laughter, and create a life I love — which is an integral part of healing and living fully; she sent me to her therapist, who lead me to another game changer and life saver — Mama Gena's School of Womanly Arts where I did all that and more. We made a follow-up appointment, but I felt better already, just knowing this.

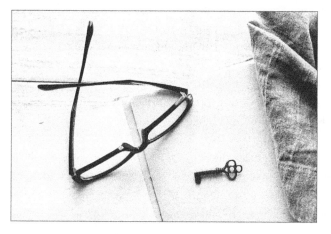

The Key to Healing is Revealed

Around that time, I went on a yoga retreat in Costa Rica with a dear friend and colleague. During lunch, a woman on our retreat was sharing how she was blown away and raving about the most powerful healing experience of her life with a breathwork rebirthing session she had with a local practitioner — she said she felt like she released a ton of trauma energy from her body.

I made an appointment right away – and that was the appointment that began the journey that saved my life.

The practitioner named Lucy spent a lot of time asking me focused questions about my past, as far back as I could remember. She was very wise, kind, and compassionate, but direct and confrontational, which is what I needed. I really did not care at this point. I just wanted to feel better and release whatever was causing my suffering.

My First Breathwork Session

She then led me through a session of continuous, conscious, connective breathing, regular and flowing, but deep, full, and circular. I eventually became semi-conscious — there, but not there. I felt all kinds of interesting sensations — I was scared about them, but she reassured me it was normal healing, to keep focused on the breathing. I felt tingling electric-like feelings in my feet, legs, arms, and hands that traveled up my body, but stopped at my chest.

It felt like a dark, black, heavy steel wall was there blocking it, making it impossible to penetrate. It felt deep and endless, like a bottomless pit. I did not like this and wanted the things I felt in my heart and chest area to go away. She lovingly said that was from my years of burying and repressing my intolerable pain. It helped and protected me as a child, but it is not serving me now.

I could release it, if I wanted.

"I can't," I told her.

She said, "Don't try. Just let it be there and breathe."

I was resisting.

She midwifed me and guided me, and I surrendered. Eventually, it literally felt like it dissolved and then the tingling and electricity traveled all over my body. Then my whole body started shaking, and I asked her what was happening.

She reassured me that it was all good — this was the trauma releasing.

"Bring it on!" I remember thinking, and it felt beyond awesome.

When that resolved, my body was as heavy as lead and I could not move, but I did not want to. I also felt the most delicious feeling of relief and lightness within me. Like hundreds of pounds of bricks of trapped trauma energy just left my body.

> *"I really did not care at this point. I just wanted to feel better and release whatever was causing my suffering."*

At the end of session, it was so powerful, I asked her what drug she just gave to me? What did she do to me?"

She said, "Nothing, that is the power of this kind of breathwork."

Now I was blown away. I knew I needed more, so she gave me the contact of a breathwork practitioner in my area, and we also continued via Skype video sessions. I traveled down to work with her in person a few more times as well. Once I brought my husband, who was enthralled with the miracles he saw in me by doing this modality, so he started doing it, too. I was saving my life — I did not care if I needed to travel, and I was grateful for credit cards.

Patsy, the woman I worked with in my area was another blessed beautiful soul, a seasoned breathworker/rebirther who has led private and large group sessions/workshops around the globe for 35 years. I was opening to a whole new world. Each session I released and healed more and more and got to deeper places. Healing is like peeling away layers of an onion, and I was committed to give it my all. It was working. Finally, something was working! I was feeling more and more at ease in my body, more and more myself.

More Release, More Healing

I did not feel done though and was frustrated. I decided to immerse my-self in a month-intensive Clarity Breathwork group program led by Dana Dharma Devi Delong and Ashanna Solaris. It was there that I released just about all of it. Billions and billions of tons of trauma energy left my body, and I knew it was gone forever, never to return.

I healed the traumatized inner child and wounded adult.

I released trauma energy from events that I did not even know were as traumatic as they were, at the time. I got clarity on many parts of my life about what happened to me, about my belief and thought patterns that governed my actions and reactions as well as the results in my life. I learned why I was triggered the way I was; why I made the adult decisions I did. I became clear that I was the only one who could heal myself, and I had the ability and innate power to do so. I had the capacity to rewrite my story, transform dysfunctional limiting beliefs and lies I had told my-self repetitively for so many years, and I freed myself from the bondage of false conditioned negative thought patterns.

"I had the capacity to rewrite my story"

Without condoning abuse and neglect, I was able to find forgiveness for all those who harmed me, as they either were ill, wounded themselves, or doing the best they could with what they knew and faced at the time. I forgave, loved and had compassion for myself and for others.

I connected to my own spirituality, to the (loving) divine in me, in each person and all that is.

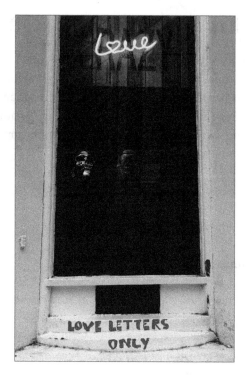

I found Gold

I found gold and I have to share it! I took the full training and got certified as a Clarity Breathwork practitioner. I took other training, growth and transformational workshops to fine tune my abilities help others heal their wounds and suffering, and get back their peace and joy.

What is revolutionary is that one key unlocks all locks. I'm going to show you what the key is that unlocks and opens the door to healing your health and wellbeing, your relationships, love life, career, how you feel inside, and ending to your suffering so everything falls into place.

This is what I want for you!

THE TRAUMA RELEASE FORMULA

The Trauma Release Formula is based on the concepts I learned when I experienced my miracle journey of trauma healing, attending and assisting at numerous healing and transformational trainings and workshops, as a Midwife, Yoga Teacher and Certified Clarity Breathwork Practitioner, and from years of helping countless others in my practice heal their suffering and get themselves back.

It is a simple five-step process:

1. Acknowledge the Trauma ⁓ *Recognize the trauma*

2. Feel the Trauma ⁓ *The healing is in the feeling*

3. Release the Trauma ⁓ *Clear your body of trauma energy*

4. Reset your central nervous system ⁓ *Allow your body to complete the instinctual trauma response cycle and resume equilibrium*

5. Cultivate Joy, Love, & Gratitude ⁓ *Create Your Authentic Life (YOU).*

It gives you a map from which to create your own releasing and resetting ritual. The goal is to reset your nervous system, get the memory of trauma out of your body, and to let your body release and clear of the trauma energy. Then you get back to yourself, can cultivate joy, and create a life you love.

What is truly mind-blowing is that there is one master key that unlocks all locks — that you can reset, release, and heal yourself and your life, to live in your joy by following these simple steps without having to spend thousands upon thousands of dollars on years in psychoanalysis, talk therapy, and medication.

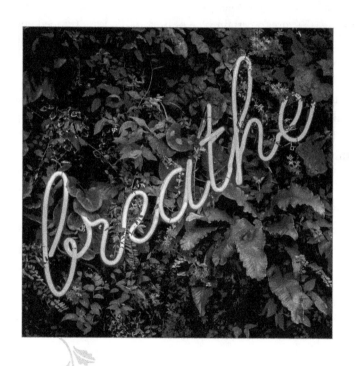

Let's discuss the one key that unlocks all locks. It is breath.

The One Key is Clarity Breathwork

Clarity Breathwork is a powerful potent healing modality, yet gentle and nurturing, that uses a certain type of breath to release trapped energy of inner stress, trauma, emotional pain and harmful repeated thought patterns from the body – resulting in lasting effective recovery.

The International Breathwork Foundation describes it: "breathwork is a dynamic body-mind practice using conscious connected breathing techniques for inner peace, enhanced well-being and personal transformation. Breathing, beyond the basic need for survival, acts as a bridge between spirit, mind, and body; between the conscious and the subconscious."

According to the foundation, "Conscious breathing is one of the quickest ways to open the heart and energize the body. When used in specific ways, breathing allows us to release and resolve emotions, belief systems, stresses and memories which are often inaccessible through the more conventional talking therapies."

Clarity Breathwork

Clarity Breathwork, a form of what was previously called Rebirthing, is a safe, easily accessible and all natural, but powerfully effective process of healing, growth and transformation that is not usually achieved with traditional therapy and modalities which only involve the logical mind. It enables you to tap into your body's tremendous capacity to rebalance and heal. It increases oxygen and energy flow in the body, helps gently release toxins, negative thoughts, inner tension and stress, suppressed wounds, painful emotions and trapped trauma within you. It leads to greater clarity, a deeper sense of knowing and profound insights into your core

life's issues. This work, and its life coaching aspects, can also bring awareness to habitual dysfunctional subconscious beliefs, repetitive patterns
and conditioning, as well as remove blocks and a sense of feeling stuck,
that limit you from living the life you want. It allows for spontaneous
completion and resolution, invites you to develop the courage to cultivate acceptance, understanding, reconciliation and even gratitude for
past hurts. It enhances love, compassion, and forgiveness of yourself and
others, and inspires you to take responsibility for your life, embrace what
is, and let go of trying to control what cannot be controlled.

> *"Wonderful inner change creates outer changes in your
> well-being, your life, your direction and sense of purpose,
> and your relationships."*

What is amazing is how it can bring consciousness to your subconscious
— which dictates much of your bodily functions, emotional responses, and behavior. Clarity Breathwork can even connect you to the spiritual realm within and around you, to reveal the true magnificence of
who you are and heal a mistaken sense of separation from these essential
components of life. The process creates an incredible feeling of relief,
aliveness, enhanced well-being, and joy. Wonderful inner change creates
outer changes in your well-being, your life, your direction and sense of
purpose, and your relationships.

How Does Clarity Breathwork Work?

❖ The Physical

Breath is what gives us life, needed fuel, energy and oxygen; exhaling
is the most effective natural detoxification. Clarity Breathwork invites
you to breathe at 100% of your lungs' capacity, accessing 100% of your
respiratory system. In modern day life, we usually breathe far less than

that, with 20-30% of our lung capacity. Oxygen is the main fuel/energy for every cell and organ in your body. During the time you are breathing completely and fully in this way, you are enabling your cells to get get fully oxygenated and energized, you are supplying yourself with maximum amount of that fuel.

You are also releasing toxins, so that your entire body can work better and operate more efficiently. Your lungs are the main organ of detoxification as well, releasing many toxins, not just carbon dioxide, so you are getting a huge cleansing and natural detoxification with breathwork. This enables your cells and organs to function most optimally and healthfully.

In the state of breathing in this way, you are bathing in healthy hormones. You are creating a more alkaline state, instead of acidic state associated with many diseases.

By doing this, everything in your body works better and more efficiently, so you are putting yourself in the most ideal state of health that is possible for you.

❧ THE EMOTIONS

Breath is also intricately involved in our emotional responses. When we are relaxed, we breathe more slowly and deeply. When we encounter a stressor, our bodies are hard-wired to go into the fight or flight stress response. Sometimes this can be lifesaving. But if there is no imminent danger, we still experience all the symptoms and effects of the stress hormones which become harmful over time, and often we are without the ability to fully process it all — especially if the stress is chronic or severe. We momentarily hold our breath, then breathe more rapidly and shallow, and the unprocessed emotions felt at the time get subconsciously repressed, and stored as trapped energy within the body, without our knowing.

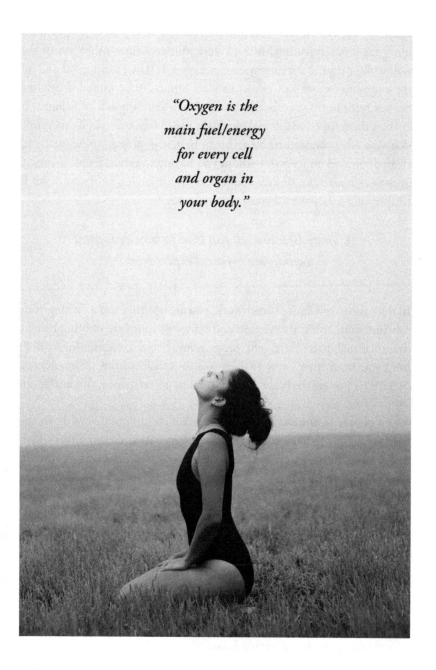

*"Oxygen is the
main fuel/energy
for every cell
and organ in
your body."*

Breath is the vehicle by which we process emotion. Clarity Breathwork puts you in a semiconscious state, gets your conscious mind out of the way so your central nervous system can reset. It is like turning off and on the computer, so we can return to ideal original state/intended original factory settings, so your body can rebalance anything out of balance. It enables the trapped emotional energy in your body and cellular memory, that was not processed to come up to be felt, expressed, processed and cleared/released on its own without you having to think, know, mentally understand, analyze, or talk about it, without having to try to make it happen or access your subconscious via thought.

> *"Clarity Breathwork can lead to transcendental and divine mystical experiences."*

In the process of Clarity Breathwork, you are opening and accessing your subconscious. You get awareness and clarity of your core limiting beliefs, dysfunctional patterning, old programming and conditioning, which frees you from them, and enables you to transform them. Breathwork literally empowers the body to reset, recalibrate, rebalance, and heal itself.

Many people in the modern world operate almost continuously in the fight or flight mode even though there is no actual danger from which to flee, wreaking havoc with their health. Animals, especially mammals, shake off trauma energy, after they escape a predator threat, and return to their normal relaxed state of being — they move on without being impacted by the trauma experience; the energy of the trauma is not suppressed, it does not build up and cause dis-ease as it does in humans. Humans tend to carry baggage of past wounds, hurts, pains, and traumas. Clarity Breathwork enables the breather to be in an altered state, so the body naturally releases this baggage of past trauma energy, and when it is released we feel better emotionally as well as physically; we are in a more optimal state of health and well-being. It is incredible to feel and to witness the immense relief that follows.

❧ Breath of Life

It even works on a deeper spiritual level, regardless of whether you believe it or not, and is inclusive of all belief systems. Spirituality means a lot of different things to different people. Whatever you believe it does not matter — God, Spirit, mother earth, goddess, the universe. The route of breath, inspire, is in spirit, which can simply be all that which transcends the body. Around the world in many cultures and religions, breath is associated with spirit, God, the infinite and eternal — from all biblical religions where God is described as breathing life into the first humans Adam and Eve, to the yogic traditions describing prana (breath) as spiritual life force energy.

The ancient yogis in the east for thousands of years spoke of prana, breath, as spiritual life force, and have used various types of breathing to creates states in the body of deep relaxation, bliss, heat, coolness, vitality/increased energy – and this is still done around the world in the modern yoga practice.

Clarity Breathwork has no association with any religion or spiritual dogma, but it sure has spiritual benefits; it enables us to explore, feel deeper into, and connect to the essence of who we are, that which is sublime and so very there, but not directly discernible through our five senses. It connects you with the less tangible transcendent aspects of you.

Clarity Breathwork can lead to transcendental and divine mystical experiences. People report they connect with a higher power, energy/presence of others who have died or are not near, but still present for reconciliation, support or guidance; they can have healing visions, access great clarity and get incredible insights.

Breathwork takes you beyond your limiting judgmental mind, beyond your body, beyond the illusion of separation from divine energy within and around us, and each other.

If you are literally taking in all this breath, inhaling the spiritual life-force fully into your being, especially with the intention to heal, the healing that takes place is all the more profound; this not only makes this modality even more compelling, but also it provides such an incredible tool, that you can access at your own will. Miracles happen.

❧ YOU CAN DO THIS!

Breathe. The full continuous breath is the main event. Breathing in this way uses the breath as a potent medicine, that has tremendous healing capacity.

It is simple and accessible to anyone who has lungs. It involves continuous, conscious, connective breathing, with a wide-open mouth and relaxed jaw, to get a full gusto inhale. To give you a sense of the ratio of inhale to exhale — it is like 3 or 4:1 but don't focus on the numbers.

Usually, it is done in savasana position/corpse pose, lying down flat in a real comfortable position using pillows, bolster, and a blanket for support and comfort. I use music, verbal supportive guidance, and gentle hands-on support during in person sessions. It can be done in water — tub, spring, lake, calm cove of sea — with a practitioner — water accelerates the process and is an awesome experience. It can be guided online as well, using Skype, Zoom or Face Time.

Inhale deep into your heart and back of your throat, like a gasp, and a soft relaxed exhale without effort or pushing, like fogging a mirror. Together, the inhale and exhale can be likened to a silent 'ah-ha.' It is circular and flowing, without pause in between. Breathing like this lasts about an hour.

❧ NO RISKS

There are no risks to breathing fully in this way, and there are no risks to feeling any emotion — all feelings are valid, holy/sacred, and safe to

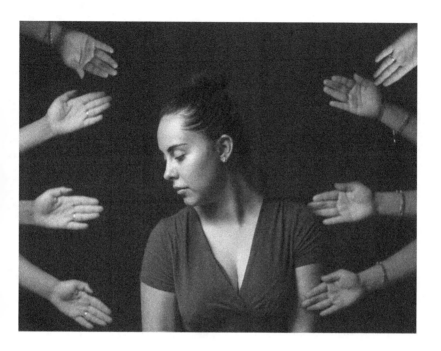

feel and express. Actually, the healing is in the feeling. All you need to do is give yourself permission to play full out and go for it, dive right in, allow and embrace all sensations as normal and healthy, what is needed to process, release and heal.

Also, there are no risks to tuning into your deepest desires, doing what you really love, what brings you real pleasure and joy as much as possible. For your higher healed self, this would never entail hurting yourself or another.

Clarity Breathwork effects are felt quickly, and they are permanent. Whatever trauma energy releases during a session, does not come back. You get up feeling healthier, mentally, and emotionally clearer and better, more spiritually connect than you already are and to that aspect of yourself.

❖ Why You Have Traumatic Responses

You have **unprocessed energy of traumas**, emotional pain and inner stress on all levels, and harmful repetitive untrue but very real thought patterns trapped in your body without the technology to release it. We live in a culture that does not understand or fully acknowledge trauma, what it is and its effect and impact on every aspect of our lives. Conventional/traditionally trained medical doctors, psychiatric and psychological therapies and even many common alternative modalities cannot help you.

Let's talk more about the stress response and research on the topic.

❖ The Stress Response

Peter A. Levine, PhD., cutting-edge trauma expert and founder of Somatic Experience for trauma healing, points out the following in his best-selling book, "In An Unspoken Voice, How the Body Releases Trauma and Restores Goodness."

Here, let's go deeper into the stress response.

Traumatic and overwhelming stressful situations of all degrees, where one feels threatened, frightened, and powerless elicits a survival instinct response, in both human beings and animals, so we can escape danger and get to safety. When animals run from a predator, they use the increased energy of the fight or flight response, to flee and protect themselves, and when free of danger, they shake and discharge the rest of it off. They involuntarily self-regulate, settle and return to their equilibrium. If the danger is imminent, with little chance of survival, the animal's trauma response is to freeze, shut down, disassociate and anesthetize, as if to play dead, which can ultimately lead to successful escape or minimize the pain of attack. Again, if the animal makes it to safety, it shakes and resets and resumes being in the calm, alert optimal state. These are universal instinctual responses of traumatic helplessness in intense overwhelming experiences of extreme danger. What is fascinating is like humans, if the animal's trauma responses are interfered with, there is usually a profound sense of defenselessness associated with increased levels of stress and fear, they can have more difficulty self regulating. Humans get stuck in a dysfunctional vicious cycle of trauma responses without the original trigger, and without resolution to completion.

Why Humans Get Struck in the Trauma Cycle

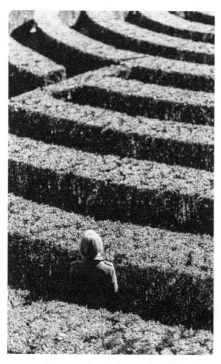

As humans, we do not often allow for our normal intuitive and primal nervous system to go through and complete this full rebound and self regulating process, and this leaves us more vulnerable to getting stuck in the trauma cycle. When exposed to reminders and events that trigger it, even when they are not considered traumatic or even upsetting to someone else, we get the fight or flight or freeze response when there is nothing to escape from — it becomes our default response to just about any stress. This takes a tremendous toll on our physical and emotional well-being.

When we are in enhanced state of arousal, we do tend to shiver, like if nervous, after giving birth, waking from anesthesia given for surgery, after shocking or terrifying news, an accident or injury, even after orgasm — but we are not taught to allow for and embrace it; rather we are encouraged to stop it, drug it, or talk ourselves out of it. Stopping it is like trying to stop a waterfall. Drugging it then makes no sense, and talking about it does not touch it — it does nothing to release the energy or reset the nervous system. When upset, stressed, or even traumatized we are taught to suppress, escape, numb, and even deny our normal reactions and feelings. This leaves us stuck physically and emotionally, which dominates our lives in many negative ways.

> *"What we resist persists, what we allow, resolves as a wave comes to a peak, then subsides. "*

Becoming aware of this normal healthy response to stress and trauma we have, lessens its gripping hold. Allowing and embracing the trauma energy and associated sensations of our reactions to emerge and complete themselves is our path to salvation and freedom from them.

✤ ACKNOWLEDGE THE TRAUMA

In my experience, one of the greatest difficulties the amazing women and men I meet is how they experience dealing with trauma — how they face their feelings and fears and feel them head on. *The healing is in the feeling, not the suppressing, denying, escaping, and numbing.* What we resist persists, what we allow, resolves as a wave comes to a peak, then subsides. It works every time and I am in awe of the power of this work.

Dive head on into it despite the resistance. It's like birth — at most intense times, women fight it, they think they can't, that something is very wrong, they are afraid of losing control and exploding. Fighting it often holds back the birth and makes it all worse, but when they are encouraged to allow, to go with the waves of sensations, and to let the sensations take over, to surrender, they birth their babies. This is the same with healing emotional pain and trauma. Often, the fear of feeling intense feelings that were never processed is harder to deal with, than feeling the actual sensation of the pain, and trauma energy itself. The panic you have about feeling the scary feelings of panic, anxiety, and emotional pain will often be your last panic attack, if you allow yourself to feel it all. No matter what type of trauma, from a horrible childbirth experience, to rape, incest, loss, abandonment, physical or verbal abuse, violence, accidents, serious illness or other acute or chronic intense stress— the trauma will stay trapped inside the body, if not released with expert care.

❧ What are Trauma Symptoms?

The symptoms you experience when the energy of inner stress, pain, and trauma is trapped in your body and your nervous system is stuck in the dysfunctional trauma response are vast, but some are listed here. With each symptom, there are many layers of potential as to what may be inside of the symptom. This revolutionary method of healing trauma will penetrate those layers, so you can heal deeply and fully. Just remember, a high impact, traumatic, or painful memory is simply that — it is an imprint of something that caused great agony, fear, and helplessness trapped into the cells and subconscious of your body. Everything that has ever happened to us is stored in our vast subconscious that governs our reactions, behavior, and lives — most of which we do have not access to, but the existence of inner stress, pain and trauma within it is causing all kinds of physical, emotional, personal and relationship imbalances; it can even cause physical and emotional dis-ease to form, so giving your attention to this healing method, will facilitate faster healing in your body and your life.

❧ 9 Symptoms of Trapped Trauma, Emotional Pain, and Inner Stress

1. You feel often stressed out, worried and anxious. This may seem like a common theme among everyone around you, but when you have endured trauma, these symptoms may be telling you to look inward and focus on what's causing your suffering.

2. You feel overwhelmed, overworked, and depleted, burned out, taking care of everyone but yourself. Often, you may even feel like you are walking around in someone's body, and not really connected to your own reality.

3. You seem to be filled with resentment, anger, rage, and other people see and notice this. The feelings of anger and rage were caused by the trauma that is now over, but much of it was repressed, and it feels as real as if the episode just happened.

4. You find that you are irritable, cranky, and reactive even to your loved ones and children. Reactions happen quick, and you wonder why they occurred. Take note: This is your wounded inner child, simply trying to get your attention.

5. You are unhappy, uninspired, unfulfilled, sad or downright depressed — you do not feel joy and this goes with you everywhere. Even when trying your best to enjoy things you used to love, like walking in the woods or a good movie, you feel no pleasure or even gloomy. This is an attachment to the imprint of trauma.

6. You are addicted to harmful habits of which you are aware, but cannot seem to stop. Harmful habits range from eating unhealthy foods, sex addiction, overwork, alcohol or drug dependence, to gambling.

7. You feel deeply embarrassed or ashamed by some part of your body. Seeing yourself in a mirror makes you cringe, and you want to cover it up, so others don't notice.

8. You may be struggling with eating disorders such as binge eating, guilt eating or not eating at all. Unhealed emotional pain, inner stress, and trauma are temporarily soothed by a bowl of ice cream, a box of cookies, or a bag of potato chips. You may even decide you just don't want food that you once enjoyed.

9. You experience brain fog and feel stuck and can't make decisions as you could in the past. You will have a thought that is severed, leaving you dazed and confused about where it came from.

These are just a few of the symptoms you may have with trapped inner stress, emotional pain and trauma, and there are many more. The trauma lives in a hidden place within your body, mind, heart and soul being. Without effective treatment, this trauma will take you a lifetime to completely heal, if at all.

I am going to give you some guidance on how you can effectively and permanently release emotional trauma from your body with ease, reset your nervous system, and get yourself back. Yes, you have to feel every sensation that may come up. Be comfortable with the uncomfortable — as there lies your freedom. But you may even find it to be fun. Choose to enjoy your healing process. Let it be easy. Once I felt I was healing, I loved and embraced every sensation that came up — "Bring it on," was my attitude, and the attitude I encourage you to have to get the best healing results. But, first I want to share a few stories about others with you.

The following includes some examples of how Clarity Breathwork has helped others in my practice. You are not alone. Many people suffer, but the good news is that you are here, and you have found the ultimate key!

First, you acknowledge the trauma, then work to release it and reset your central nervous system to go on to heal, and experience joy again.

While I have helped thousands of people on their healing journey, here are just a few short stories so you can see what is possible for you.

Dad Finds His Joy and Becomes Pain Free

I worked with a dad who had previously hired me help him and his wife birth two of their babies. He was having marriage problems. He was unhappy, struggling and unable to express his feeling or feel intimacy. He was not enjoying sex on a deeper level and he was way too overprotective with his children. When he was a child, he had a nanny who sexually abused him for years. He never told anyone, not even his wife or parents. The nanny had threatened him and told him that his parents would never believe him. He really didn't think anyone would believe him and he stuffed his feelings; at age 40, he was tired of suffering and ready to do the work.

He was in physical pain as well. He had chronic inflammation in major joints, and none of the multiple medical and holistic providers he had consulted had been able to help him. It impaired his ability to work, exercise, and impacted his personal life. After a series of Clarity Breathwork sessions, he released the trauma and emotional pain trapped in his body, and all of the joint pain went away. It's important to note that our mind and body are intricately connected and Clarity Breathwork healed something that no other practitioner or modality could heal!

He forgave his parents and told his mother, who did believe him and support him. While his father was deceased, he was able to visualize a reconciliation with his dad for closure. While not condoning his abuse, he let the toxic energy of the nanny go; he acknowledged that she was either severely ill, disturbed, abused, or wounded herself.

After Clarity Breathwork, he felt more at ease, relieved, and got his joy back which improved his marriage and deepened their relationship. He even became more connected to his children and loosened up his overprotective grip on them. He became renewed, lighter, more playful and loving. He was grateful to be alive and for all the blessings in his life.

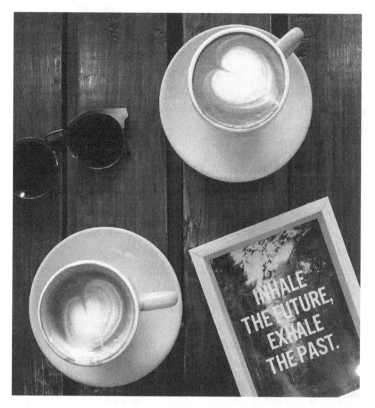

A Return to Trust and Joy

I helped a woman who suffered with depression, anxiety, insomnia, acid reflux, and migraines. Nothing was working for her. She felt stuck in a bad marriage and was afraid to leave because of her children. When she was a child, she had a little sister who was born with Down Syndrome. She loved her little sister, but at age 4, she was told the baby had died. Thirty years later, she found out her parents had lied to her and that her sister was alive and had been placed in an institution. Not only did she suffer from the loss of her little sister, her family buried their own depression and inability to cope with her sister's condition, had lied to her and she felt betrayed.

During a series of Clarity Breathwork sessions, she released the trauma energy and deep pain of it all, forgave her parents, and no longer felt depressed or anxious. Now she is doing what she loves, feels better, and sleep better without any migraines. She is now visiting her sister weekly and is very close to her. Her marriage is on the mend, and she is focused on it with more clarity, love, compassion, transparency, and is more tuned into her family.

Healing Birth Trauma

I worked with a woman who was an admitted work-alcoholic. She was exhausted, overweight, worried, stressed to the max, ashamed of her body and found herself eating more and more. Nothing she did was ever good enough. She was trying to keep it all together. She was working two full-time jobs, and taking care of her only son, who was on the autistic spectrum — which started a day after a routine vaccine. She felt she had failed at natural childbirth when a nurse told her that she was not trying hard enough and was not coping well, so she gave up and ended up with a C-section. The anesthetic did not work so she felt and screamed during the agony of the surgery until it was too much to bare — and then they gave her so much drugs, she needed a respirator to breathe. With all the medications she was given, she was was too drugged to hold her baby right after birth. She was traumatized and terrorized by her experience, so she never had another child. She blamed and loathed herself because she really wanted to have more children.

During Clarity Breathwork, she released the birth trauma energy, envisioned giving birth naturally and saw herself holding her newborn baby as soon as he was born. She imagined healing her cesarean scar and breathed out the trauma, pain, grief, and anger of raising an autistic son. She reconnected with her spirituality and is loving herself with compassion. She is allowing herself to feel more, embrace her emotions, let go of one of her jobs, and now finds time to relax and even play. Her marriage has improved, she is eating more healthfully and returned to her normal weight.

Trauma manifests in many ways. It may be expressed by emotional pain, inner stress, physical problems, illness, or relationship and life issues. Trauma can exist in the body, even if there doesn't appear to be any history of physical, sexual, or verbal abuse.

❧ SUMMARY OF SOME SYMPTOMS

To summarize some of the symptoms caused by trapped trauma and emotional pain, many people say they are:

• Stressed out, worried and anxious

• Overwhelmed, overworked and depleted, burned out,
  taking care of everyone but themselves

• Filled with resentment, anger, rage

• Irritable, cranky, and reactive;

• Unhappy, uninspired, unfulfilled, sad or downright depressed –
  do not feel joy

• Addicted to harmful habits and do not do much to take care
  of themselves

• Embarrassed or ashamed by some part of their body

• Struggling with eating disorders

- Stuck and can't make decisions

- Disconnected from themselves and others

- Shut down, powerless without a voice

- Longing for something more and better, but don't even know what they want, or thinking something outside of them will rescue them and make them happy

- Plagued with self loathing, self doubt, not feeling valued, worthy or good enough, like a failure

- Filled with shame, blame or a sense of being wrong

- Lonely and isolated — without community, or even within their circle of friends and family

- Sensually and sexually shut down and turned off

- Troubled by relationship issues

- Battling career and work problems

- Suffering with ongoing physical symptoms or chronic health conditions from body aches and pains, to migraines, intestinal issues, acid reflux, trouble sleeping, high blood pressure, heart disease, autoimmune disorders, cancer …the list goes on.

If you can relate or have some of these feelings or issues, you are in the right place.

❧ CLARITY BREATHWORK IS FOR YOU:

- If you have any of the feelings or issues I mentioned in this book, or as I and my clients did;

- If you have physical or emotional symptoms that modern medicine, or other modalities can't diagnose or heal;

- If you experienced trauma of any kind, emotional pain, or inner stress that impacts your life today;

- If you feel stuck in your life, have what feels like emotional blocks, negative self talk, or habitual behavior that limits you;

- If you want healthy natural ways to reduce inner stress, heal from emotional pain and trauma in a way that lasts;

- If you want increased energy, vitality, to feel like yourself again;

- If you want more ease, flow and joy in your life and relationships;

- If you have physical and emotional problems that have not been responding to the various treatments and therapies you have tried;

That you have not been able to heal, and feel stuck in making progress in your life, are often because these main causes have not been addressed at all.

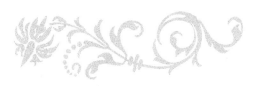

The Root Cause

The surface level issues you are suffering with are not the source, the root cause. You have unprocessed energy of traumas, emotional pain and inner stress on all levels since birth and early childhood onward (possibly even before that — while in the womb), and harmful repetitive untrue but very real thought patterns trapped in your body without the technology to release it.

We live in a culture that does not understand or fully acknowledge trauma, what it is and its effect and impact on every aspect of our lives.

Conventional/traditionally trained medical doctors, psychiatric and psychological therapies and even many common alternative modalities can not help you.

*"Your world is a reflection
of your internal self."*

❧ SUBCONSCIOUS/UNCONSCIOUS MIND

Most of our thoughts and behavior are governed by our subconscious/unconscious mind. Our conscious mind that we have access to is only the tip of the vast consciousness iceberg beneath. Everything that has ever happened to us, including our core self limiting beliefs, repetitive patterns and conditioning that produce results in our lives, is recorded and contained in our sub/unconscious mind – like a highly sophisticated computer. Your world is a reflection of your internal self.

We attract, interpret/project and manifest – set up situations in our lives to what fits our belief system – most of which is subconscious. We got stuck in past traumas without even knowing it. We act out untrue beliefs to prove them true, project them onto everyone/everything or overcompensate and do anything to prove it wrong/isn't true.

☙ It's Not Your Fault

While it is not your fault how you were born and conditioned and patterned to believe, and what happened to you as a child, and most of what we face in life that is not in our control – it is your responsibility to liberate yourself if you want to heal and be free, and enhance all aspects of your life – including work and relationships with others.

Maybe all these therapists, doctors, conventional and alternative modalities were not able to help you....but there are effective revolutionary tools and I'm going to show you how they work so you can apply them in your life.

By now you understand that those problems that have been getting in the way of your wellbeing and living, keeping you from your most healthy, fulfilled, joyous, life, great loving relationships, keeping you from showing up fully in your personal life and your work often have the same underlying causes.

Many of your multiple problems are from trapped energy in your body of unprocessed trauma, emotional pain, inner stress and repetitive dysfunctional and false thought patterns.

You've read my story and you've read some stories of other people, how that happened for them...you can begin to imagine what the possibility is for you. There is hope!

START YOUR OWN HEALING PLAN

Dance those Traumatic Memories OUT!

I want to invite you to tap into your joy, your play, your aliveness, even your sensuality and sassiness — all an integral part of healing and living fully. For those of you who do not know me — I love to dance.

❧ DANCE

Dancing is a shortcut to creating your happy. It's contagious. It is a great way to relieve stress and it can easily transform energy of feeling stuck, in a funk, or bad mood into joy.

❧ DAILY PRACTICE

It's my daily practice — I do it everywhere: at home with my kids cooking and cleaning, at work with clients and colleagues, offices, stores and markets, busy city street corners and crosswalks, with people in labor all hours, home or hospital, I have assisted many moms to dance their babies out. I've been to multiple trauma and healing, growth and transformation workshops and trainings with 10,40, 100, 500, 2500 people feeling, expressing, moving through and dancing the full range of human emotions — grief, anger, exuberance, sensuality, creating energy, wild fun and play.

Indigenous cultures around the world and throughout history used music, vocalization and movement to feel, express and move emotion in community – joy, celebration, as well as grief and rage.

❧ LET IT OUT

As babies and toddlers, little boys and girls, we authentically, innocently, proudly had raging temper tantrums to feel, express, move through

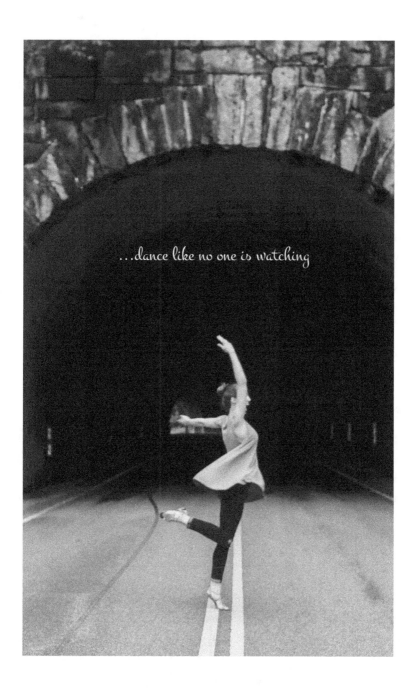

...dance like no one is watching

sadness and anger — screamed; we sobbed, writhed around, stomped, banged, pounded and kicked. We released, reset, then got up and went back to playing. When we were excited and joyous we skipped, danced, sang and shouted with glee just the same. When full of stress we played harder, got rowdy, climbed the walls, and moved the energy. When were we told to shut down, tune out, turn off, disembody, and disconnect from ourselves, keep it in? When were told feeling sad or anger is wrong? When we told not to express how we feel? When were we told being happy is bad too? When did we stop loving ourselves and others like we did as babies? Babies/toddlers do not doubt their magnificence, they are total love, comfortable and proud being themselves, they know they are awesome, beautiful, lovable, worthy, and valued.

❧ Hope

There is hope. WE CAN absolutely TRANSFORM THIS as adults.

SO – I invite you to get more into your body, out of your mind, and let the words and beat move you, however, it does, wherever it takes you.

❧ Go Deep

Go deep. Explore how you feel, express, and you are your emotions with music and dance, vocalize if needed — get into it, let it all go and dance like no one is watching. Start in your a private room in your home, just dim the lights and blast the music. Soon, you will feel more and more at ease with it. Then once you are comfortable try it at work or just about anywhere, really.

❧ Channel Your Inner Child

Channel your little girl/boy comfortable in your body, innocently, authentically, proudly even sensually expressing and being themselves. If it feels silly and awkward, then you're going in the right direction. Even though there is no wrong, right, mirrors, performance, video – fire the inner critic. It's something to cultivate if not used to doing for a while, but your body already knows. I have been doing it for years. If you need guidance, you can watch others dancing with passion on dance videos or in my group events for a moment, but I really want to encourage you to explore you.

SO let's get down! Push your edges, growth is always beyond the comfort zone.

✤ Move, Dance, Feel

Dance your emotions, feel and move them through your body. Feeling, expressing and moving the energy of emotions through your body is a big component of the healing, and then creating happy energy and life.

Make a playlist of songs that are sad, angry, loving and then upbeat. Commit to a time that works for you each day. Play four types of songs: 1 or 2 songs each. Get into the music, go out of your thinking mind, and go deep within, explore the way your body naturally feels, moves, and expresses the full range of emotions through music and dance.

Play a really sad song ⌒ feel the song, the words, the grief, sob, roll around the floor and let the music reach your soul and move your body spontaneously and even sensually through the sadness.

Play a really angry song ⌒ feel the song, the words, and have a full blown temper tantrum ⌒ stomp or writhe around the floor, roar/scream/curse, push/press against a wall, stagger, crawl, kick and punch a cushion/pillow/sofa/yoga bolster, bang a pillow, or belt against the floor or sofa.

Play a love song ⌒ imagine singing it to yourself caressing every part of your precious body, hug yourself and sing it to you as if you were singing it someone you love with all your heart and soul — like your child, your inner child. If you want to — play with your inner sensual self, move nice and slow, mindfully — you can massage yourself naked with scented almond or coconut oil.

Play an upbeat happy song ∼ shake, move, do hip and head circles. There are so many choices to songs here — pick what makes YOU feel good, vibrant, fully alive, sexy and sensual.

Always end with the love song and upbeat song, so you don't get stuck in the muck. But let the dancing tell your story, express your feelings, and the joy you want to create.

Some of the most powerful methods to compliment healing trauma and emotional pain, in addition to breathwork and body movement — is freeform writing, journaling your feelings, and transformative exercises.

THE POWER OF WRITING AND JOURNALING

Affirmations and Self-Talk

Scientific research tells us we have 50,000 to 70,000 thoughts per day, and most are unconscious — imprints/ patterns/old programing, non-verbal and childhood memories from birth, early childhood, family and cultural conditioning. For every self-limiting thought you notice that proceeds emotional pain — write it down and consider how it is not true at all. Write the opposite of that thought and feel that to be more true. For example, if you think "I am not good enough" — note the complete opposite, write and imagine what it FEELS like to say "I am good enough, I am perfectly imperfect just as I am and I am doing the best I can'" and sit with that.

If you think "I am damaged from trauma and will never heal" simply turn that around to "I am not damaged, and I can fully heal." Ponder how it feels to tell yourself lies that make you suffer, or truths that empower or make you feel well.

❧ LIMITING BELIEFS TO CHANGE

Here are some common limiting beliefs you can work with to practice. Remember change the negative language to positive, empowering language:

• I am not safe, it's not safe to be here

• I can't trust anyone

• I am separate and alone

• Pleasure or love leads to pain

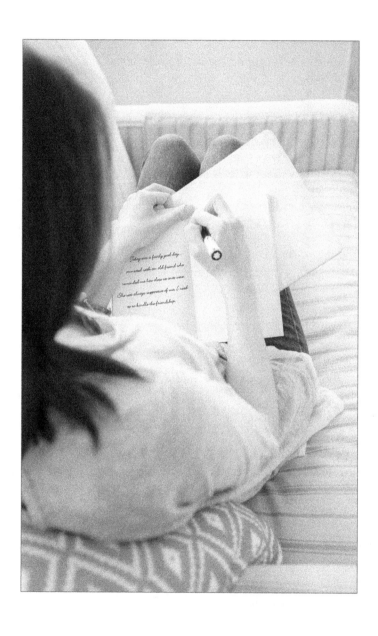

- Life is hard or a struggle

- I am wrong or never good enough, they are wrong or not good enough

- It's all my fault, it's all their fault

- I hurt people or people hurt me

- I can't make it without pain or difficulty

- No one loves me/I am not lovable or wanted, something is wrong with me

- I'm too this or that

- Nothing is working or works for me

- I don't want to be here

Once we release the trapped trauma and thought energy causing our dis-ease and suffering, part of this work is realizing most of thoughts we think over and over again, the beliefs we came to believe about ourselves are not really our own, and they are not true at all.

What we concentrate on expands – energy flows where the mind goes (negative low vibration thought limits us and creates negative results, positive higher vibration thought creates expansive enhancing results in our lives).

When we become aware of this, they have less and less power over us, and we have the ability to decide what thoughts we want to believe, how we can change them and decide to think them repetitively instead of the habitual self-sabotage, there is transformation.

Also, when we let out the trauma/negative thought energy, transmute our stories of limitations, there is huge relief, freedom and space, and part of this work is tuning into our inner wisdom, what we really feel, love, deeply desire, and are passionate and enthusiastic about, and then living from that place; we find our truth, our gifts, our purpose, and we can more effectively manifest what we want to attract and create in our life — and then do our part to make it happen.

When we are aligned with who we really are, lit up, turned on, and excited about living and doing what we truly love and came here to do, we bring ourselves and others higher; when we are not, we bring ourselves and others down.

❧ Free-flow Writing and Journaling

I highly recommend free-flow writing and journaling, or making art of your feelings. Create a running super-journal of your journey. The Journey Journal will help you document emotional triggers, create forgiveness, get clarity, and heal the experience.

Here are some helpful guided practices as well.

❧ How to Cultivate Daily Joy

You can create a daily cultivation of joy. Write 10 things you love about yourself, 10 things you are or did that you are proud of, 10 things for which you are grateful, 10 things you deeply desire, that you would love being, doing or having — each with one or two steps in the direction of manifesting and making it happen. Track your results. Note your shifts, how you are feeling, progress over time — 1 week, 1 month, 3 and 6 months, 1 year. You will be amazed by the results of this inner work. It is one of the most effective, yet simple things you can do to help heal your mind, body, and soul. Joy creates more joy. It is that simple.

Journal Notes

Turn to

Back of

Book & Begin

Your Journal

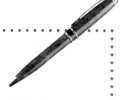

Write,

Draw,

Stamp…

…whatever
moves you!

❧ WRITE LETTERS

Write an angry letter to someone who you feel has hurt you. Let it out — all what you would say if you had your voice, what you could not say at the time. Burn or shred it.

Write a second letter to that younger you, of loving comfort and compassionate support, giving him or her coping tools and wisdom that you did not have then.

Write a third letter back to you, imagining from that person what in his or her higher fully evolved self would say to you if he or she knew what you felt. Write a forgiveness letter back to that person, from your higher self, without condoning harmful behavior — to free yourself from the poison. You are free to keep this private…but consider sharing it with the perpetrator and how that would help you heal.

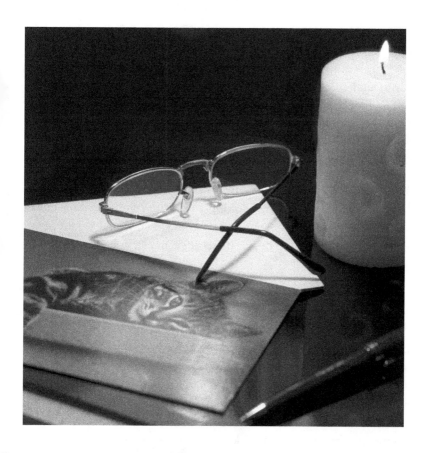

Let it out

START YOUR OWN DAILY HEALING PROCESS NOW

You can start now to formulate your own daily rituals which create new habits, and new pathways in the brain and nervous system. Use the methods and tools described here, you can use to begin your healing journey. Get started. But first Breathe.

❧ YOUR NEXT STEPS

You can feel, dance, move, write, and journal yourself into joy, peace, hope, and gratitude, but you need to work with someone who can help you release the trapped energy inside your body. If you would like to work with me in a group or private setting, contact me.

❧ TAKE THE NEXT STEP TO HEALING

We have talked about how to release trauma and discussed some ways you can help yourself start the healing process with breathing, movement, writing, and other exercises. If you would like to take this further and do deeper work, I want to share with you how to turn this immediately useful information into lasting healing and transformation. There are tools, training and support for you!

I want to encourage you to work with someone to help you get the healing results you need, so you can return to living a healthy, joyful life.

These are the steps you need to take to get the results that are possible for you whether you do it with me or with another practitioner who has similar training and does similar work.

Know your strength. You are stronger than you realize.

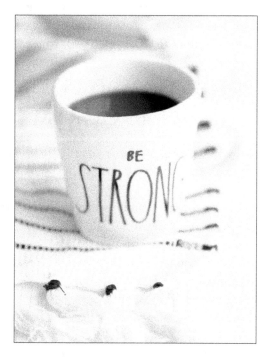

❧ Do Breathwork

Commit to yourself and a series of 10 breathwork sessions.

Healing is a journey, not accomplished by just one breathwork session, especially if you have years of suffering with emotional pain, physical problems, long standing life problems, past chronic ongoing or intensive trauma — but this is the quickest most effective and lasting way, at least for me and countless others around the world, and does not require years of expensive extensive psychoanalysis and therapy, diagnostic testing and treatment.

**I am giving you an invitation to join me in my upcoming program
I created - the rebirth yourself VIRTUAL program that is a
series of 10, 2-hour group online sessions and want to take
a few minutes to show you how it works.**

REBIRTH YOURSELF
VIRTUAL PROGRAM™

The Rebirth Yourself Program is available virtually, in group or VIP private session packages. It is designed to give you the tools to:

1. Heal your emotional wounds and traumas in a way that lasts (to feel like yourself again- or even better!).

2. Reduce inner stress and feel incredible relief, lighter and more comfortable in your body.

3. Feel increased aliveness, energy and vitality, and have more ease and flow in your life.

4. Remove what feels like immovable blocks, transform self limiting beliefs, thought patterns and behavior that stand in your way to living the life you want.

5. Have greater clarity, a deeper sense of knowing and profound insights into your core life's issues, decisions, and unique gifts.

6. Cultivate acceptance, understanding, reconciliation and even gratitude for past hurts - and see the gifts in your story.

7. Enhance forgiveness, compassion and love for yourself and others.

8. Take responsibility for your life, your inner joy and peace - no matter what challenges you face.

9. Connect to your spirituality, with the true magnificence of who you are, your bigger purpose and vision for your life; restore your self-worth and value in this world.

10. Connect to and feel the benefits of a community, develop deep lasting authentic friendships with others who are going through similar experiences of healing from pain, transformational growth, and reclamation of joy.

❧ REBIRTH YOURSELF VIRTUAL GROUP PROGRAM™

Say YES to yourself! I'm ready to take down what's holding me back from living the happy, fulfilled, and abundant life that is my birthright with the **Rebirth Yourself Virtual Program**™

Begin reclaiming your inner calm, joy, fulfilled, and abundant life right away!

Contact me for more information about scheduling your sessions.

I invite you to step up. Here is the link:
http://homesweethomebirth.com/rebirth-yourself

Register now and get started on your healing journey today.

I can't wait to work with you and for you to feel huge healing and transformation in your life — The miracles I myself have experienced and witnessed. When I think about my decision point in my life every day, I am brought to tears with gratitude.

In the modern world where it has never been acceptable to fully feel and express the full range of emotions, being REAL, transformational healing and living in full joy are revolutionary acts. The mission of the Rebirth Yourself Personal Program is to empower you to heal from inner stress, pain, and trauma that has held you back in all aspects of your life, live in relaxed state of joy and fulfillment, and healthy emotional expression safe for all —in the world that urgently needs us to heal, bring ourselves and others higher, and show up fully with our gifts. Let's heal and learn to let ourselves shine together!

FIVE TOP QUESTIONS ASKED ABOUT CLARITY BREATHWORK AND TRAUMA RELEASE

I know you are feeling fear and hesitation because I and other have felt it. I want you to know this work CHANGED AND SAVED my life and I want this for you too. Let me answer the top five questions people ask me before jumping in and then if you have further questions, you can always contact me directly.

☙ I am Afraid

1. I am afraid of my pain, to revisit the past and my trauma. If you reading this book and perhaps filled out surveys and attended one of my webinar trainings you are in some degree of pain and suffering. First of all you are in good hands — I have either felt, or seen it all as human being, midwife, and Certified Clarity Breathwork Practitioner, have healed myself and have helped others heal. No emotional pain is too big or dangerous — I know what darkest and lowest is all too well, 10 on a scale of 1 to 10, I have been there, and came out on the other side from this work only.

I tried it all as I told you. This work is completely safe without risks, other than healing, feeling so much better beyond your wildest imagination, back to yourself if you can remember what that was like, in delicious relief, joy and calm, creating a life you love. What could be better?

We live in a culture that is not comfortable with discomfort and pain, and encourages escape, denial, keeping it in, or numbing. Pain calls us to listen for the messages, to take important action. Your body does not lie. Pain is indeed inevitable, but suffering, how we react and the stories we tell ourselves about the sensations we feel, is optional. In this world, there is sun and rain, light and dark, joy and pain. They are all needed, essential to living and are all sacred/holy essential parts of our being. Feeling all feelings leads to living fully in our greatest potential.

When doing this work, the invitation is to allow, love and embrace all sensations and feelings, even if it seems at times — especially early on, not comfortable or downright overwhelming. "Bring it on," is the ideal mindset, as there lies your freedom.

Stay present and open and curious but the main thing is, dive right it, let it all be as it is, but most important, is to keep breathing.

Know you are safe and supported and loved by those who support and love you — including your spiritual guide(s). I am there with you, holding space, guiding and supporting you but I do not try to fix, change, or suppress you — as that interferes. You can draw on unseen or your own internal support. You are stronger than you think. You have the innate power to heal yourself, if given the opportunity, and the tools. YOU are bigger than any pain, fear, or memory.

What events occurred in the past, passed, and is not happening now. What is happening are results of your trapped pain and trauma. Your recurring self-limiting thought patterns are robbing you of your present. The healing and transformation is in the feeling, letting go, surrendering and trusting the process, your body's infinite wisdom to process, reset and release what is not serving you.

All is confidential — we create boundaries — we all agree what goes on in the private or group sessions stays in the sessions.

As in the heat of birth (a normal and healthy huge transformation), during the most intense sensations of late labor and as baby is crowning/emerging, many women tell me they can't, it is too much, they want a cesarean, they think something is really wrong, they panic, think they will explode, go crazy, even die, and they tend to fight it. It is when they are reassured all is well, reminded to tap into their strength they did not know they had, they pray to a higher power, stop resisting, let go and surrender to the brilliant process far wiser than any human, go with and ride the waves, that they give birth. Every time. The same happens in breathwork sessions, healing andrebirthing.

Resistance is common and means you are going in the right direction. If you start thinking this isn't working, I don't like it, it's too hard, I am not doing it right, it is easier to just stay where I am/what I'm used to — even if your life is not working, you feel terrible suffering and dis-ease — welcome it, know those are all signs to keep on going, keep breathing. What you resist, persists, and only increases your suffering.

⤋ No time, No money

2. I don't have the time or money; I'm too busy; and I can't afford it. I felt that way, too, before I took the initial leap and invested in my healing. It was about what was my priority. I made time and money for what I valued, and this was a necessity for me. What I am aware of from reading all of my client surveys is the extent of pain you feel and its impact on your life, that two hours once a week or every other week times 10, and even with a ritual self care practice daily — is like a blip in the scheme of things.

If I added up the years, the energy, everything I spent on all sorts of treatments, therapies, and remedies with all sorts of providers and therapists, plus the books, workshops and retreats — it is overwhelmingly huge; how do you measure the cost, the time and energy of terrible suffering, the inner pain and torture, not feeling fully alive and well, life and relationship problems, self sabotaging and limiting myself, and getting in my own way?

Let me ask you, what is it costing you in time, money and energy, your peace of mind, joy, fulfillment, relationships, work/career by not doing this? How much time, money, energy, vitality and opportunity do you lose daily, weekly, monthly, yearly by not healing and continuing to suffer with this pain and inner stress you have had for years that you told me about in the survey or did not tell me about.

Let me tell you — the way I feel now is priceless, I would have paid anything and spent whatever the time/energy needed had I known about it sooner.

When I look back at my decision to make the investment for my own Clarity Breathwork, it was beyond worth every dollar, every minute; I am just so grateful/thankful to my younger self she had that courage to make that decision. Because of her I am back to myself, healed fully, living in my inner calm and joy, so full and fulfilled I am able to give back and help you and others birth and rebirth themselves and have that same experience. That is what I want for you.

✦ HELP!

3. What if I need personal help, how will I get that in an online group session? I thought that too, but some of my most powerful healing sessions were in a group. There is an option for private sessions — I did and felt I needed both, but most do just fine in group sessions. And many benefit immensely by private sessions. There are centers all over the world sometimes as common as yoga studios, where people go to breathe in a group regularly. The benefits of a group are many — knowing you are not alone can help heal the wound of illusion of separation; hearing, and witnessing others' experiences can help validate your own and you realize your pain/divinity in others/their pain and divinity in yours; the universality of pain and wounds comforts as you see what you feel how you reacted to what you faced is normal and more common than you imagined; knowing we are all in this together is also comforting; if anyone needs help, speak up and let me know, I am there with you throughout;

we all hear and see each other, the support and guidance I give to one can apply to all of you so let it in, and see how it benefits you. If something releases from one of you, it heals and releases from all. Receiving support like honest loving feedback and observations can accelerate your growth and transformation.

Connecting in conscious supportive loving community to people like yourself, where vulnerability and authenticity is the norm, often begins in the relationship with a professional practitioner; it can lead to profound healing — some of my greatest of friendships that last to this day are from those I met and connected with in my group workshops.

There is plenty of opportunity to maintain this connection on the private Facebook group and beyond — you get out of it what you put in to it.

I also do have a spiritual perspective and trust that we are all held and supported, we call on support of our guides, mentors, our biggest support staff alive or not, angels, the divine I trust we are held by the beloved, and supported, that nothing will come up that you (or I) can not handle. And again, you can opt for private one-on-one sessions.

❖ Can I Really Do This Work?

4. Some say "Anne, what if I don't trust myself to do the work?" If you don't trust yourself to get on a two-hour group online session one time a week or every other week for 10 weeks, and follow my guidance, then this program may not be for you or you may not be ready to heal and transform your life. But, if you are ready to have healing breakthroughs, and this is calling you, plow through your resistance. Resistance as I said is a great sign and I will welcome it and you where you have my individualized and undivided attention.

❧ WILL THIS REALLY WORK FOR ME?

5. A common question I get and I had myself was what if it doesn't work for me? I tried so many things and nothing helped. Nothing works for me, why would this? Another is, I do breathwork exercises in yoga, or I have done rebirthing before and didn't like it.

Nothing will work for me is a limiting untrue thought; the opposite is usually more true — what if it does work for you? Try that on and imagine how it feels if it does work for you? Imagine what it feels like to heal, to not have your suffering, to feel joy and relief and calm? To love your life?

There are no guarantees to anything, but again, I also tried just about everything and nothing worked before for me either, but this worked for me completely and has lasted to this day, as I told you: it saved my life and so many others I have witnessed. This is powerful work like no other I had experienced.

It is not at all yoga pranayama breathing exercises, which are wonderful and have their place; this is a specific form of breathwork to heal trapped energy of inner stress, dysfunctional repetitive thinking, pain, and trauma.

I do not know what type of breathwork you did, and what training your practitioner had, or what support was given. This is a unique revolutionary approach an art and science, that works for those who are ready and eager to do it, to play full out. The only thing in your way is yourself. We often get in our own way. It is time for healing, freedom, and joy!

Invitation to Learn More...

I invite you to step up. Here is the link:
http://homesweethomebirth.com/rebirth-yourself

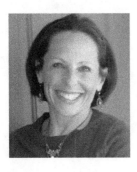

About the Author

ANNE MARGOLIS
CNM, LM, MSN, BSN, RNC

Anne Margolis is a Licensed Certified Nurse Midwife, Certified Yoga Teacher, and Certified Clarity Breathwork Practitioner. She is a third generation guide to mamas birthing babies in her family. Anne has helped thousands of families in her 22+ year midwifery practice and has personally ushered the births of more than 1000 healthy babies into the world. She has also guided countless human beings to heal from emotional pain, inner stress and trauma, and reclaim their joyfulness, calm, and overall sense of well-being.

Through her online childbirth course "Love Your Birth," her online and in-person midwifery for pregnancy and postpartum support consultations and care, her birth professional mentoring, her holistic gynecology and Clarity Breathwork offerings, she infuses wisdom, compassion, inspiration, and joy into the entire process of healing and wellness.

Anne is a two-times Number One international best-selling author. Anne's work, insights, and advice have been seen on local, national, and international radio programs, and TV shows and movies including four episodes of "A Baby Story," on TLC Discovery Channel, the award-winning feature documentary, "Orgasmic Birth," and "The Human Longevity Project."

Anne has also been a featured speaker and expert panelist at distinguished events for Weil-Cornell School of Medicine, the University of Pennsylvania School of Nursing, RCC State University of New York School of Nursing, and Birthnet Association of Childbirth Professionals and Hudson Valley Birth Network to name a few.

Anne's Clarity Breathwork groups have been hosted at several yoga studios and wellness centers, including the conscious, high vibration and transformational community at The Assemblage in New York City. Anne is a proud founding member of The Health and Wellness Business Association, which was created to promote initiatives that support better collaboration, interaction and ethical business practices within the health and wellness business community.

Learn more now and get started on
your healing journey today.
http://homesweethomebirth.com/clarity-breathwork-new-york

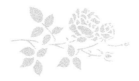

References
Dana Delong, Peter Delong and Ashanna Solaris "Clarity Breathwork Training Manuals Levels 1-4" ClarityBreathwork.com , 2018.

Peter Levine, PhD., "In an Unspoken Voice: How the Body Releases Trauma and Restores Goodness." North Atlantic Books, 2010.

Journal Notes

Journal Notes

Journal Notes

Journal Notes

Journal Notes

Journal Notes

Journal Notes

Journal Notes

Journal Notes

Journal Notes

Journal Notes

Journal Notes

Journal Notes

Journal Notes

Journal Notes

Journal Notes

Journal Notes

Journal Notes

Journal Notes

Journal Notes

Journal Notes

HOME SWEET HOMEBIRTH MIDWIFERY, PLLC
DISCLAIMERS AND POLICIES
AFFILIATE and PROMOTION DISCLAIMER

The following information is disclosed by Home Sweet Homebirth Midwifery, PLLC ("we" or "us") to you in accordance with the Federal Trade Commission's 16 CFR, Part 680 and 698: "Affiliate Marketing Rule." Sections of this book or website www.homesweethomebirth.com (the "Site") may allow you to purchase products and services online provided by other third party merchants. Some of the links that we post on this Site or book are "affiliate links." This means that if you click on the affiliate link and purchase an item through that link, that we will receive an affiliate commission. For example, we are a participant in the Amazon Services LLC Associates Program, an affiliate advertising program designed to provide a means for us to earn fees by linking to Amazon.com and affiliated sites.

We are not responsible for the quality, accuracy, timeliness, reliability or any other aspect of the products and services purchased through affiliate links, the information contained on third party sales page, or any other third party links, products or services we promote. In addition, the merchant for your purchase will have privacy and data collection practices that are different from ours. If you make a purchase from a merchant on their website or on a website that we have promoted or posted a link to on any of our online medium, the information obtained during your visit to that website or that merchant's online store, and the information that you submit as part of the transaction, such as your name, e-mail address, street address, telephone number, and credit card number, may be collected by that merchant. For more information regarding any merchant, its' online store, its' privacy policies, or any additional terms and conditions that may apply to your visit of its' website, visit that merchant's website and click on that merchants relevant pages and their informational links, or contact that merchant directly.

You release us and our affiliates from any damages that you may incur, and agree not to assert any claims against them or us in connection with your purchase or your use of any of the products, services, or information contained on sales page made available to you by third parties through our Site or promoted on any of our online medium. Your participation, correspondence or business dealings with any third party found on or through our Site or promoted on any of our online medium, regarding payment and delivery of specific goods and services, and any other terms, conditions, representations or warranties associated with such dealings, are solely between you and that third party. You agree that we will not be responsible or liable for any loss, damage, or other matter of any sort incurred as the result of any third party transaction.

TESTIMONIAL DISCLAIMER

The following information is disclosed by Home Sweet Homebirth Midwifery, PLLC ("we" or "us") to you in accordance with the Federal Trade Commission's 16 CFR, Part 255: "Guides Concerning the Use of Endorsements and Testimonials in Advertising." Testimonials appearing in this book or website www.homesweethomebirth.com (the "Site") are received via text, audio, or video submission. They are individual's actual experiences, reflecting the real life experiences of those who have used our products and/or services. We do not claim that they are typical results that consumers will generally achieve. The testimonials are not necessarily representative of all of those who will use our products and/or services. We are not responsible for any of the opinions or comments posted to this Site. You understand that any testimonials or endorsements (herein "Opinions") by our customers or audience represented on this Site, or through our products, programs, other websites, content, landing pages, sales pages or offerings, are solely opinions from individuals. Similarly, any information contained on this Site and on our other programs, content and offerings are solely our opinion and therefore, not representations, warranties, or guarantees of any kind.

WELL BEING DISCLAIMER

This book or website (www.homesweethomebirth.com (the "Site") is for informational purposes only. Home Sweet Homebirth Midwifery, PLLC ("we" or "us") and our subsidiaries, owners, principals, directors, executives, employees, staff, or agents are only licensed health care providers or professionals in their state and/or area of expertise. The information contained on this Site will not treat or diagnose any disease, illness, or ailment and if you should experience any such issues you should seek the advice and examination of your registered physician or practitioner as determined by your own judgment. You understand the information contained on this Site is not a substitute for health care, medical or nutritional advice of any kind. You understand and agree that you are fully responsible for your well being, including your dietary, mental and physical choices and decisions and that of your child. You agree to seek medical advice as determined by your own judgment before taking any action in connection to the information contained on this Site or discontinuing use of any medications as prescribed by your medical practitioner. We shall in no event be held liable to any party for any direct, indirect, punitive, special, incidental or other consequential damages arising directly or indirectly from any use of this material, which is provided "as is", and without warranties. Your continued use of the site indicates your acceptance of the terms and modifications or future modifications.

REFUND POLICIES

All discounted bulk packages and programs are refundable within 30 days of the date of purchase, only 10 business days prior to start of program, less a 10% reversal fee. After that period, the fee is not refundable. There are no refunds on online courses or services that provide access to online documents and videos. There are no refunds for services already rendered. There is a 48 hour business day cancellation policy for private sessions, unless there is an emergency: you are fully responsible for payment of single sessions canceled less than 48 hour business days from date of scheduled appointment and will not receive a credit towards another session if you purchased a package. There are no refunds for missed prepaid private appointments canceled within 48 business day hours of the missed appointment; if there was an emergency, credit will be given towards another same form of appointment. Should you prepay for a series of sessions or appointments and then decide to cancel future appointments, there are no refunds. There are no refunds for purchasing a series of breathwork sessions or yoga classes (like a yoga class card) that you missed or did not complete, and there is no credit for missed group sessions.

CPSIA information can be obtained
at www.ICGtesting.com
Printed in the USA
BVHW040839030919
557434BV00009B/88/P